CHAIR-ASSISTED PELVIC FLOOR STRENGTHENING

Your comprehensive guide to regain core strength after pregnancy with chair exercise and pelvic floor stretch

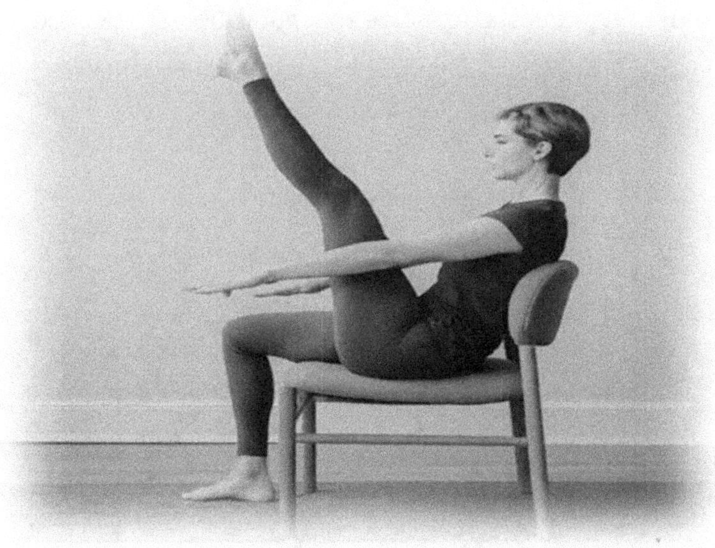

MARTINE J. TOLEDO

1

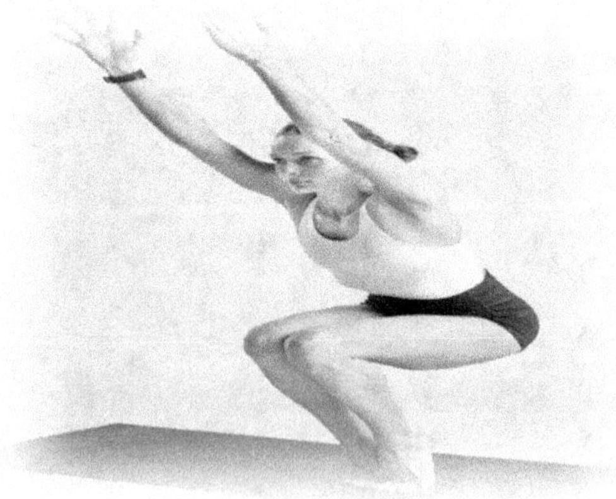

TABLE OF CONTENT

INTRODUCTION

Sam was a creature of habit. Routine ruled his life, much like the dust bunnies accumulating under his sofa. His days were a monotonous blur of work, takeout dinners, and evenings spent slumped on the couch, flipping through channels. He felt sluggish, ached constantly, and at 42, already resembled a deflated balloon more than the vibrant young man he once was.

One rainy afternoon, boredom finally won over inertia. He wandered into a dusty bookstore, drawn by a faded sign promising "Wellness Within Reach." There, nestled amongst self-help manuals and dusty biographies, he found your book. Its colorful cover and title - "Unleash Your Inner Dynamo: Rediscovering Health through Simple Steps" - piqued his curiosity.

He hesitated, the book feeling oddly heavy in his hand. But something, a flicker of hope, urged him to buy it. That night, curled up under a worn blanket, he began to read. Your words, filled with empathy and practical advice, resonated with Sam. He learned about the connection between movement and energy, the power of nourishing food, and the importance of sleep. It wasn't magic, but a call to action.

The next morning, Sam felt a spark. He dusted off his sneakers, a relic from his forgotten exercise days. He cooked a simple, vibrant meal from your recipe suggestions. The taste buds he thought long-dormant danced with flavor. That night, sleep came easier, leaving him refreshed and energized.

Days turned into weeks, weeks into months. Sam embraced your simple steps. He took brisk walks, savored healthy meals, and prioritized proper sleep. The pounds slowly melted away, replaced by a newfound confidence. He joined a gym, discovering the joy of movement. His laughter echoed through the house, replacing the silence of neglect.

One day, looking in the mirror, Sam no longer saw a deflated balloon but a man with a twinkle in his eye and a spring in his step. He wasn't just healthier; he was happier, more alive. Your book, a chance encounter in a dusty bookstore, had become a catalyst for transformation.

Sam's story, dear reader, is just one of many. Your words have the power to ignite change, to rewrite narratives, and to unleash the inner dynamo within us all. So, keep writing, keep inspiring, and let the ripple effect of your words continue to transform lives, one story at a time.

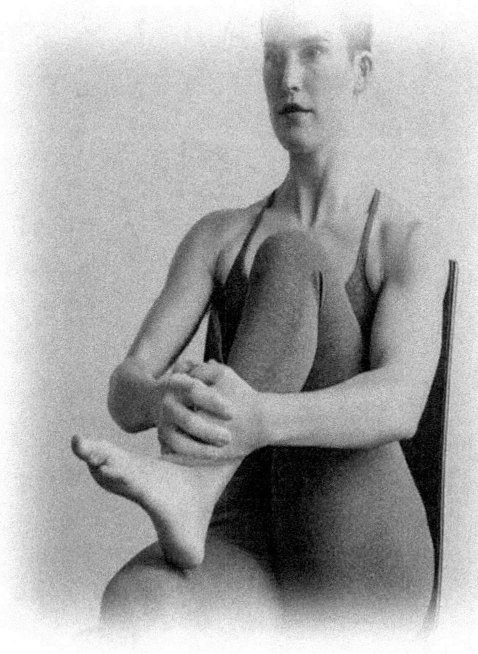

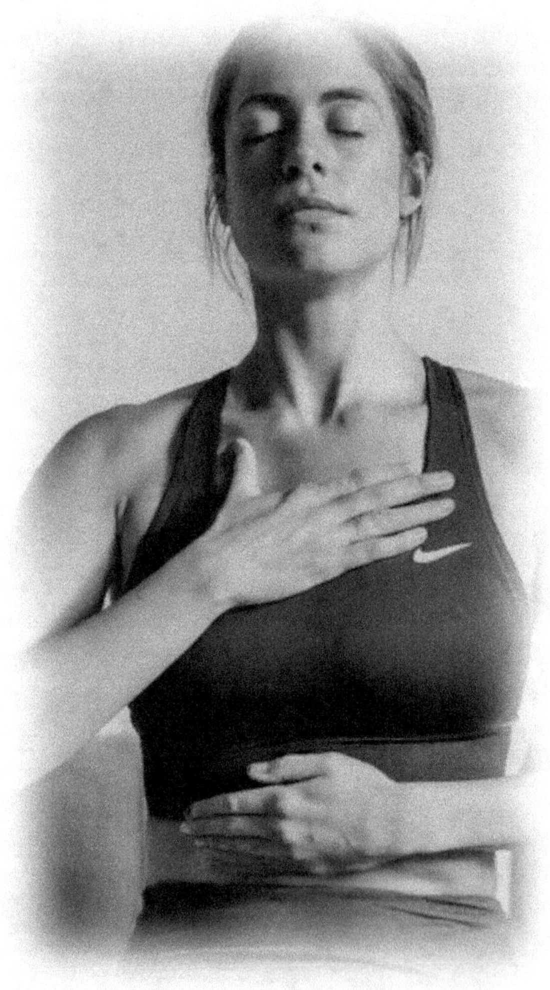

What are Pelvic Floor Muscles and why are They Important?

Beneath the surface, deep within your pelvis, lies a group of muscles often referred to as your "hidden powerhouse." These are your **pelvic floor muscles**, and they play a critical role in various aspects of your health and well-being. Let's delve into what they are and why they deserve your attention:

Understanding the Pelvic Floor:

Imagine a hammock made of muscles spanning the base of your pelvis. This hammock supports several vital organs, including your bladder, uterus (in women), rectum, and small intestine. The pelvic floor muscles act like a sling, providing crucial support, controlling various bodily functions, and contributing to core stability.

Key Functions of Your Pelvic Floor:

- **Bladder and Bowel Control:** These muscles act as gatekeepers, preventing involuntary leakage of urine and stool. Weak pelvic floor muscles can lead to incontinence.

- **Sexual Function:** They contribute to sexual pleasure and arousal in both men and women by influencing blood flow and sensation.

- **Core Stability:** They work synergistically with other core muscles to support your spine and improve posture, balance, and even athletic performance.

- **Pregnancy and Childbirth:** During pregnancy and childbirth, these muscles undergo significant stress and stretching. Strengthening them beforehand aids in recovery and reduces the risk of complications.

Why Should You Care?

Strong pelvic floor muscles are essential for numerous aspects of your life. They can:

- **Prevent incontinence:** Leakage of urine or stool can be embarrassing and affect quality of life.

- **Enhance sexual function:** Stronger pelvic floor muscles can lead to stronger orgasms and better sexual experiences.

- **Improve core strength and stability:** This can benefit your posture, balance, and even athletic performance.

- **Aid in pregnancy and childbirth:** A strong pelvic floor can assist in supporting your growing baby and potentially reduce the risk of complications.

- **Boost overall health and well-being:** Strong pelvic floor muscles contribute to a healthy pelvic ecosystem, potentially impacting bladder, bowel, and sexual health.

Remember: Your pelvic floor muscles are often neglected, but taking charge of their health through exercises like those outlined above can reap numerous benefits and ensure a strong foundation for your overall well-being.

Benefits of Chair-Assisted Strengthening

Chair-assisted pelvic floor strengthening exercises offer a convenient and accessible way to improve the health and function of these crucial muscles. Here are some key benefits you might experience:

Enhanced Bladder and Bowel Control:

- Reduced risk of urinary incontinence (leaking urine during activities like coughing or sneezing)

- Improved bowel control, potentially reducing fecal urgency or leakage

- Increased confidence and improved quality of life due to better control over your bodily functions

Improved Sexual Function:

- Heightened sensation and pleasure during sexual activity

- Stronger orgasms for both men and women

- Enhanced sexual function after childbirth for women

Strengthened Core and Stability:

- Improved core strength and stability, leading to better posture and balance

- Reduced back pain and risk of injury

- Enhanced athletic performance

Additional Benefits:

- Potential reduction in pelvic organ prolapse (dropping of pelvic organs due to weak muscles)

- Improved pregnancy and childbirth experience

- Increased overall pelvic health and well-being

Convenience and Accessibility:

- Chair-assisted exercises require minimal equipment and space, making them perfect for busy individuals or those with mobility limitations.

- They can be easily incorporated into your daily routine, even while sitting at work or watching TV.

Gentle and Effective:

- Chair-assisted exercises offer a low-impact option, making them suitable for beginners or individuals with certain health conditions.

- They allow for gradual progression and customization to match your fitness level and needs.

Holistic Approach:

- Strengthening your pelvic floor can positively impact various aspects of your health and well-being, creating a ripple effect of benefits.

Remember: Consistency is key. Regularly performing chair-assisted pelvic floor exercises can lead to significant improvements in your pelvic health and overall well-being.

For a personalized approach, consult with a healthcare professional or pelvic floor therapist to create a customized exercise program to address your specific needs and goals.

Who Can Benefit from this Program?

Chair-assisted pelvic floor strengthening exercises offer a wide range of benefits and can be suitable for many individuals. Here's a breakdown of who can particularly benefit from this program:

Individuals Seeking to Improve Pelvic Floor Function:

- **People experiencing urinary incontinence or leakage:** This program can help strengthen the muscles responsible for bladder control, potentially reducing or eliminating leaks.

- **Individuals with bowel concerns:** Strengthening your pelvic floor can improve bowel control and potentially alleviate issues like fecal urgency or leakage.

- **Women experiencing symptoms after childbirth:** Childbirth can impact pelvic floor strength. These exercises can help regain strength and potentially address issues like prolapse or diastasis recti.

- **Individuals seeking enhanced sexual function:** Stronger pelvic floor muscles can contribute to stronger orgasms and a more fulfilling sexual experience for both men and women.

Those Looking for a Low-Impact Exercise Option:

- **Individuals with limited mobility or joint pain:** Chair-assisted exercises provide a gentle and effective way to strengthen your pelvic floor without putting stress on your joints.

- **People recovering from surgery or injuries:** These exercises can be tailored to fit your recovery needs and gradually improve pelvic floor strength without strenuous activity.

- **Busy individuals:** The exercises require minimal equipment and space, making them easy to incorporate into your daily routine even with a busy schedule.

Other Groups Who Can Benefit:

- **Athletes:** Strong pelvic floor muscles can improve core stability and potentially enhance athletic performance.

- **Pregnant women:** Strengthening your pelvic floor can support your growing baby and potentially make childbirth easier.

- **Older adults:** As we age, pelvic floor muscles weaken, increasing the risk of incontinence. These exercises can help maintain strength and prevent future issues.

Important Note: While chair-assisted pelvic floor exercises are generally safe and beneficial for many individuals, it's important to consult with a healthcare professional before starting any new exercise program, especially if you have any underlying health conditions or concerns. They can help you determine if this program is right for you and recommend any necessary modifications.

Remember, taking charge of your pelvic floor health can have a significant impact on your overall well-being. Chair-assisted exercises offer an accessible and effective way to strengthen these important muscles and reap the numerous benefits they provide.

- Disclaimer and Safety Information

Disclaimer and Safety Information for Chair-Assisted Pelvic Floor Strengthening

It's crucial to provide clear disclaimers and safety information before suggesting any exercise program, particularly one focused on a sensitive area like the pelvic floor. Here's a comprehensive disclaimer you can adapt for your content:

Disclaimer:

The information presented in this program is intended for educational purposes only and should not be construed as medical advice. It is always recommended to consult with a qualified healthcare professional, such as a doctor or pelvic floor therapist, before starting any new exercise program, especially if you have any pre-existing medical conditions, injuries, or concerns. They can assess your individual needs and recommend a safe and appropriate exercise plan for you.

Safety Information:

- **Listen to your body:** Stop any exercise that causes pain or discomfort.

- **Start slowly and gradually increase intensity and duration:** It's important to progress gradually to avoid straining your muscles.

- **Maintain proper form:** Ensure you perform the exercises correctly to avoid injury. Consider seeking guidance from a healthcare professional or qualified instructor for proper form technique.

- **Respect your limitations:** Don't push yourself beyond your capabilities. Modify exercises as needed and focus on proper execution rather than quantity.

- **Be mindful of personal health conditions:** If you have any pre-existing conditions, discuss this program with your healthcare professional before starting. Certain exercises may not be suitable for everyone.

- **Seek professional help if needed:** If you experience any pain, discomfort, or worsening symptoms, consults your healthcare professional immediately.

Additional Notes:

- This program is not a substitute for professional medical advice or treatment.

- Individual results may vary depending on factors like body composition, fitness level, and adherence to the program.

- Consistency is key for optimal results. Integrate these exercises into your routine for long-term pelvic floor health benefits.

By incorporating this disclaimer and safety information, you can help ensure that your audience understands the importance of consulting with a healthcare professional and prioritize their safety while performing these exercises.

Understanding Pelvic Floor Activation: You're Key to Strength

The pelvic floor muscles are often referred to as your hidden powerhouse, yet understanding how to activate them can feel like a mystery. Worry not, for this section guides you towards mastering your pelvic floor activation!

Imagine your pelvic floor as a hammock:

This hammock supports vital organs like your bladder, uterus (in women), and rectum. By activating the muscles in this hammock, you strengthen its support and unlock benefits across various aspects of your well-being.

Feeling the Activation:

Unfortunately, unlike flexing your bicep, feeling your pelvic floor muscles engage can be more subtle. Here are some tips to guide you:

- **Imagine stopping your urine midstream:** Although not recommended to practice consistently, visualize tightening the muscles you'd use to do so. You may feel a subtle lift or squeeze sensation internally.

- **Focus on the "Lift" not the "Squeeze":** Think of pulling your pelvic floor muscles upwards and inwards towards your belly button, not just squeezing them together.

- **Engage, Hold, Relax:** Practice short tensing and relaxing cycles to understand the sensation. Start with brief holds of 3-5 seconds and gradually increase over time.

Remember:

- **Don't hold your breath:** Breathe normally throughout the exercises.

- **Activate, not Contract:** Avoid clenching your buttocks or abdominal muscles; the activation should primarily be internal.

- **Consistency is Key:** Regular practice, even just a few minutes daily, leads to stronger and more responsive muscles.

Finding the Flow:

Once you grasp the activation techniques, try incorporating them into daily activities. Imagine engaging your pelvic floor while:

- Standing up from a chair

- Coughing or sneezing

- Lifting objects

Beyond Activation:

While activation is crucial, consider seeking professional guidance from a physiotherapist or pelvic floor therapist. They can assess your individual needs, offer personalized exercises, and address any specific concerns you might have.

Remember, understanding and activating your pelvic floor muscles is an empowering journey towards improved core strength, bladder and bowel control, and overall well-being. Start exploring, listen to your body, and unlock the power within!

Breathing Techniques for Optimal Pelvic Floor Engagement:

Proper breathing plays a vital role in effective pelvic floor activation and exercise execution. Here are some key techniques to remember:

Diaphragmatic Breathing:

- This is the ideal breathing pattern for pelvic floor exercises. Place your hands on your stomach. Inhale slowly through your nose, feeling your belly expand outward. Exhale slowly through pursed lips, feeling your belly draw back in.

- Practice diaphragmatic breathing independently before incorporating it into your pelvic floor exercises.

Breathing Coordination:

- **Exhale during activation:** As you perform a pelvic floor squeeze, exhale slowly and steadily. This creates downward pressure on your pelvic floor, enhancing activation.

- **Relax on inhale:** Inhale smoothly as you release the pelvic floor squeeze. Avoid holding your breath.

Additional Tips:

- **Maintain a relaxed posture:** Avoid hunching or tensing your shoulders.

- **Breathe naturally:** Don't force your breath; focus on smooth and natural inhales and exhales.

- **Practice makes perfect:** Regularly practicing diaphragmatic breathing will make it easier to coordinate with your pelvic floor exercises.

Benefits of Optimal Breathing:

- Enhances relaxation and reduces tension, creating a better environment for pelvic floor activation.

- Improves core stability and coordination, which can benefit overall exercise performance.

- Assists in maintaining proper form during pelvic floor exercises.

- Importance of Consistency and Progression

Consistency and Progression: You're Keys to Unlocking Powerful Pelvic Floor Muscles

When it comes to strengthening your pelvic floor muscles, two principles reign supreme: **consistency and progression**. Just like building any muscle group, achieving optimal results requires dedication and strategic planning. Let's explore why these principles are crucial for your success:

Consistency:

- **Think "marathon, not sprint":** Aim for regular, daily practice, even if it's just a few minutes. Just like watering a plant daily is more effective than a weekly drenching, consistent activation keeps your pelvic floor muscles engaged and responsive.

- **Make it a habit:** Integrate short exercises into your routine. Do them while brushing your teeth, watching TV, or waiting in line. Consistency trumps intensity in the long run.

- **Celebrate small wins:** Every squeeze, hold, and lift contributes to your progress. Acknowledge your effort and stay motivated!

Progression:

- **Challenge yourself gradually:** Once your muscles feel comfortable with an exercise, gradually increase the duration, repetitions, or difficulty level. Introduce variations or add resistance with light weights or bands.

- **Listen to your body:** Pushing too hard can lead to fatigue or injury. Stop if you feel discomfort and adjust the exercise or take a break.

- **Track your progress:** Keep a log or use an app to record your sets, reps, and any modifications. Seeing your progress can be incredibly motivating.

Remember: Consistency and progression work hand-in-hand. Consistent practice ensures progress isn't lost, while gradual challenges keep your muscles stimulated and growing stronger. Here are some additional tips:

- **Combine exercises:** Aim for a diverse routine that includes exercises targeting different muscle groups and movement patterns.

- **Seek guidance:** Consult a healthcare professional or pelvic floor therapist for personalized recommendations and progression advice.

- **Be patient:** Building strength takes time. Don't get discouraged if results aren't immediate. Celebrate every step towards your goals.

Top Tips for Success with Chair-Assisted Pelvic Floor Strengthening:

Mindset:

- **Embrace the journey:** Remember, this is a process, not a quick fix. Be patient, motivated, and celebrate even small improvements.

- **Focus on quality over quantity:** It's better to perform a few exercises correctly than many with poor form.

- **Listen to your body:** Stop if you experience pain or discomfort, and consult a healthcare professional if needed.

Technique:

- **Master the activation:** Ensure you understand and correctly activate your pelvic floor muscles before proceeding with exercises.

- **Coordinate your breath:** Exhale during activation and inhale as you relax. Maintain smooth, natural breathing throughout.

- **Focus on form:** Pay attention to proper posture and avoid engaging other muscle groups unnecessarily.

Routine:

- **Find your rhythm:** Integrate exercises into your daily routine at a convenient time, even if it's just a few minutes each day.

- **Incorporate variety:** Choose different exercises from the program to target various muscle groups and movement patterns.

- **Track your progress:** Keep a log or use an app to monitor your sets, reps, and modifications. Seeing progress can be motivating.

Additional Tips:

- **Make it fun:** Listen to music, watch TV, or engage with a supportive friend while exercising.

- **Seek professional guidance:** Consult a healthcare professional or pelvic floor therapist for personalized advice and exercise variations.

- **Join a community:** Look for online forums or support groups to connect with others on their pelvic floor health journey.

- **Invest in supportive resources:** Consider purchasing pelvic floor-specific exercise equipment or apps for guidance and tracking.

- **Remember, consistency is key!** Regularly practicing these exercises will yield the best results in the long run.

By following these tips and remaining committed, you can successfully utilize chair-assisted pelvic floor strengthening exercises to improve your pelvic health, core strength, and overall well-being. Remember, you are not alone on this journey!

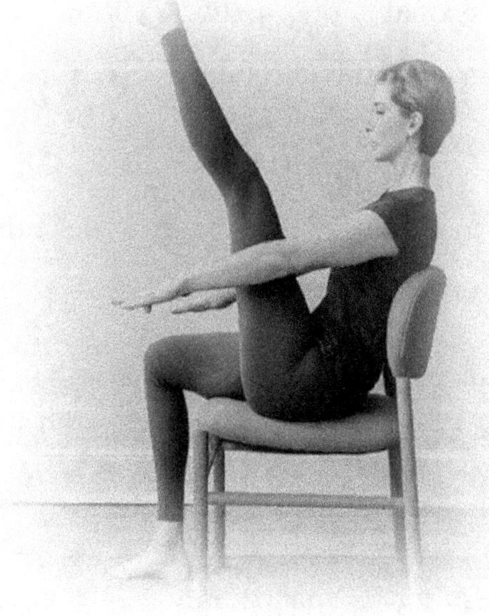

CHAIR-ASSISTED

EXERCISES:

1. SEATED SIDE BENDS:

Introduction: This exercise targets the oblique's, which indirectly support the pelvic floor and improve core stability.

Instructions:

- Sit upright in a chair with your back straight and feet flat on the floor.

- Inhale and reach your right arm overhead, reaching with your left hand towards your right hip. Engage your core and imagine lifting your pelvic floor as you reach.

- Exhale and return to the starting position. Repeat on the other side.

- Continue for 10 repetitions per side.

Illustration:

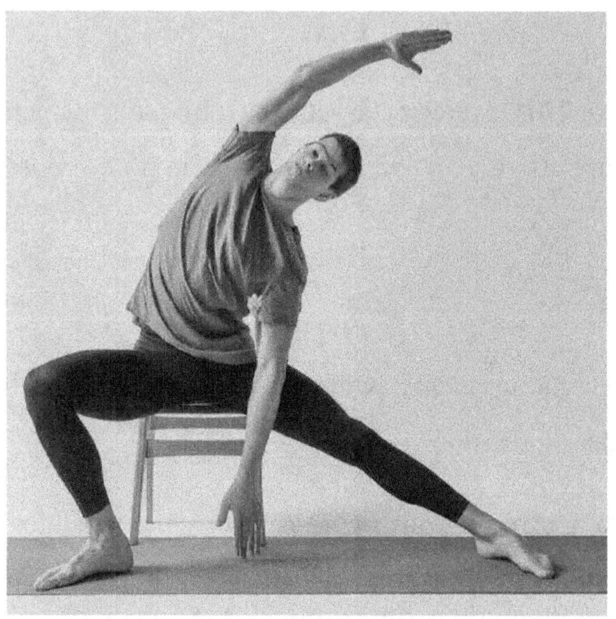

Benefits: Strengthens oblique's, improves core stability, activates pelvic floor muscles.

Tips: Don't slouch or twist your spine. Keep your core engaged throughout the movement.

Sets & Reps: 3 sets of 10 repetitions per side.

2. CHAIR SQUATS:

Introduction: This classic exercise works multiple muscle groups, including the glutes, hamstrings, and core, which indirectly support the pelvic floor.

Instructions:

- Stand in front of a sturdy chair with your feet shoulder-width apart and toes slightly pointed outwards.

- Slowly lower your body as if sitting back into the chair, keeping your back straight and core engaged.

- Push through your heels to return to standing, squeezing your glutes at the top.

- Repeat for 10-15 repetitions.

Illustration:

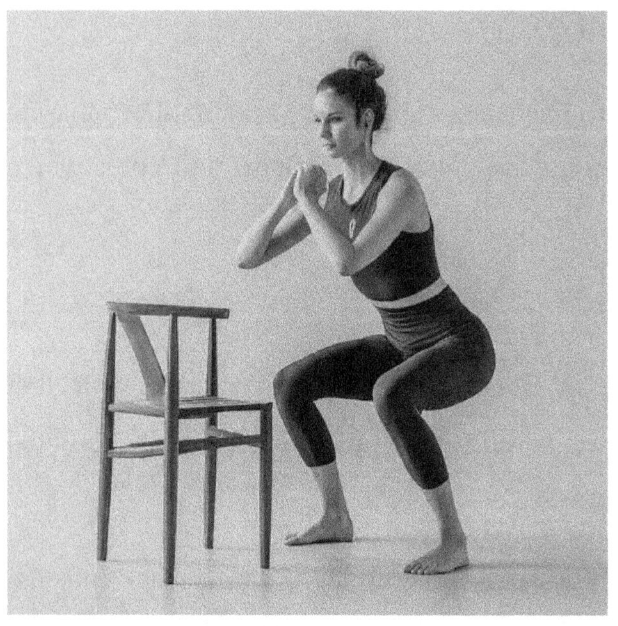

Benefits: Strengthens glutes, hamstrings, and core, improves balance and coordination.

Tips: Don't let your knees cave inwards. Keep your back straight and core engaged throughout the movement.

Sets & Reps: 3 sets of 10-15 repetitions.

3. SEATED CAT-COW:

Introduction: This gentle exercise helps mobilize the spine and indirectly activates the pelvic floor.

Instructions:

- Sit upright in a chair with your hands resting on your thighs and knees bent.

- As you inhale, arch your back slightly, looking up and dropping your shoulders. Engage your core and imagine lifting your pelvic floor.

- As you exhale, round your back, tucking your chin to your chest, and drawing your belly button inwards.

- Continue for 10 repetitions.

Illustration:

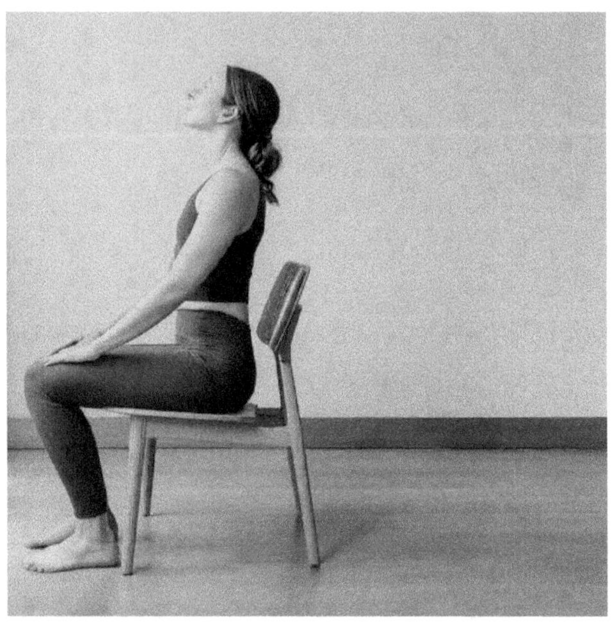

Benefits: Improves spinal mobility, relaxes muscles, activates pelvic floor indirectly.

Tips: Breathe deeply and smoothly throughout the movement. Don't force any movements that cause discomfort.

Sets & Reps: 3 sets of 10 repetitions.

4. ARM CIRCLES:

Introduction: This exercise promotes circulation and indirectly activates the pelvic floor by engaging core muscles.

Instructions:

- Sit upright in a chair with your back straight and arms out to the sides at shoulder height.

- Make small circles with your arms, first forward for 10 repetitions, then backward for 10 repetitions.

- Focus on engaging your core muscles throughout the movement.

Illustration:

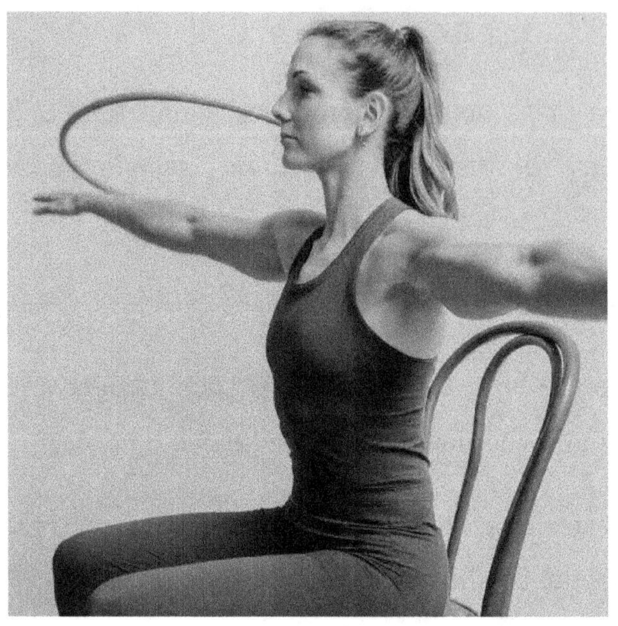

Benefits: Improves circulation, activates core muscles indirectly, and enhances coordination.

Tips: Keep your back straight and shoulders relaxed. Breathe normally throughout the movement.

Sets & Reps: 3 sets of 10 repetitions per direction.

5. DEEP BREATHING:

Introduction: While not technically an "exercise," deep breathing plays a crucial role in proper pelvic floor activation and relaxation. This is not intended to be the only exercise in your program, but can be incorporated before or after other exercises.

Instructions:

- Sit upright in a chair with your back straight and eyes closed.

- Place one hand on your belly and the other on your chest.

- Inhale deeply through your nose, feeling your belly expand first, then your chest .as you breathe in. Exhale slowly through your pursed lips, feeling your belly draw back in first, then your chest.

- Continue for 5-10 minutes, focusing on your breath and relaxing your body.

Illustration:

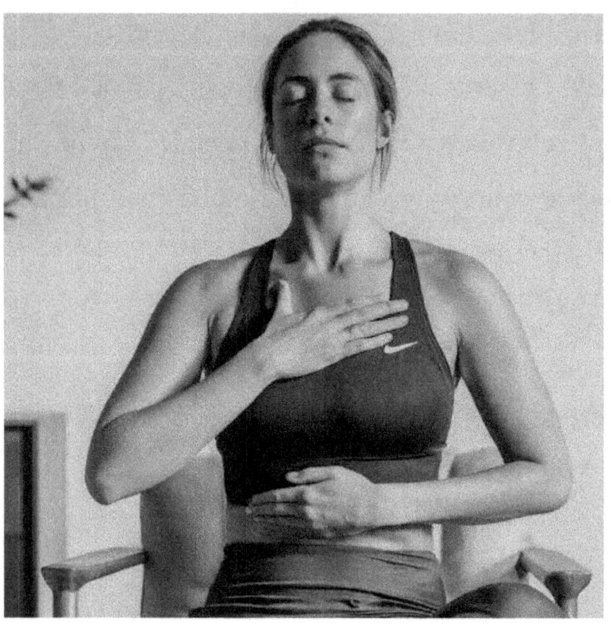

Benefits: Reduces stress and tension, improves relaxation, and prepares body for pelvic floor exercises.

Tips: Focus on your breath and avoid forcing anything. Don't judge yourself; simply observe your breath.

Sets & Reps: As needed, can be done before or after your other exercises.

6. SEATED LEG RAISES WITH HIP SQUEEZE:

Introduction: This exercise strengthens the inner thighs and hamstrings, indirectly supporting the pelvic floor.

Instructions:

-Sit upright in a chair with your back straight and knees bent.

-Engage your core and lift one leg up, keeping it straight. As you lift, squeeze your inner thighs and pelvic floor muscles simultaneously.

-Hold for 3-5 seconds, and then slowly lower your leg back down. Repeat with the other leg.

-Continue for 10-15 repetitions per leg.

Illustration:

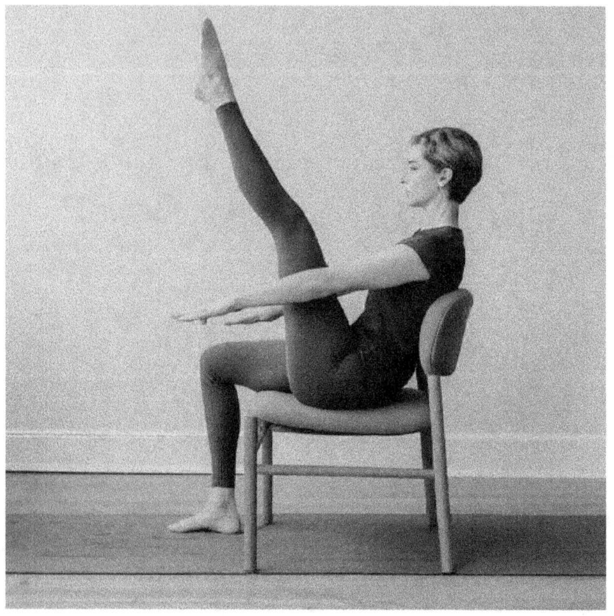

Benefits: Strengthens inner thighs and hamstrings, activates pelvic floor, and improves balance and coordination.

Tips: Keep your back straight and core engaged. Don't lift your leg too high.

Sets & Reps: 3 sets of 10-15 repetitions per leg.

7. SEATED RUSSIAN TWISTS:

Introduction: This exercise works the oblique's and core, indirectly supporting the pelvic floor and improving stability.

Instructions:

-Sit upright in a chair with your back straight and knees bent. Lean back slightly, engaging your core, and lift your feet off the ground.

-Rotate your upper body from side to side, reaching with your hand towards the opposite hip as you exhale. Engage your pelvic floor with each twist.

-Continue for 10-15 repetitions per side.

Illustration:

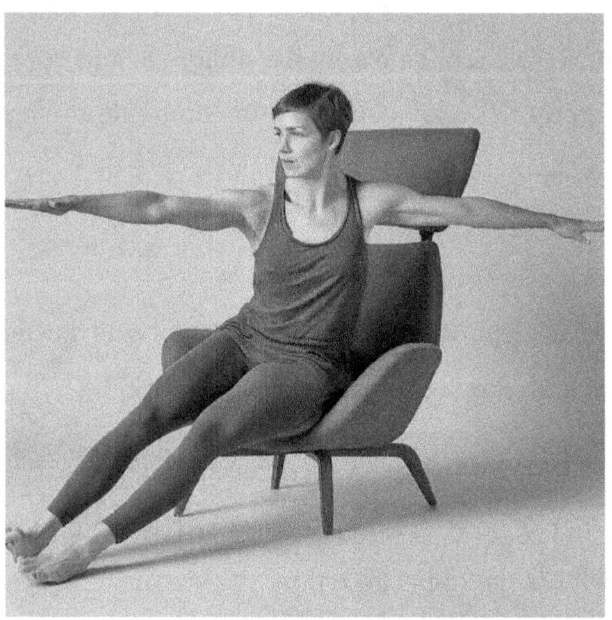

Benefits: Strengthens oblique's and core, improves stability and coordination, activates pelvic floor indirectly.

Tips: Keep your back slightly reclined and core engaged throughout the movement. Don't twist your spine excessively.

Sets & Reps: 3 sets of 10-15 repetitions per side.

8. MARCHING IN PLACE WITH KNEE LIFTS:

Introduction: This exercise incorporates cardio and strengthens the quadriceps and core, indirectly promoting pelvic floor **health.**

Instructions:

-Stand in front of a sturdy chair with your hands lightly resting on the back for balance.

-March in place, lifting your knees high towards your chest while engaging your core and pelvic floor muscles.

-Continue for 30-60 seconds, maintaining a comfortable pace.

Illustration:

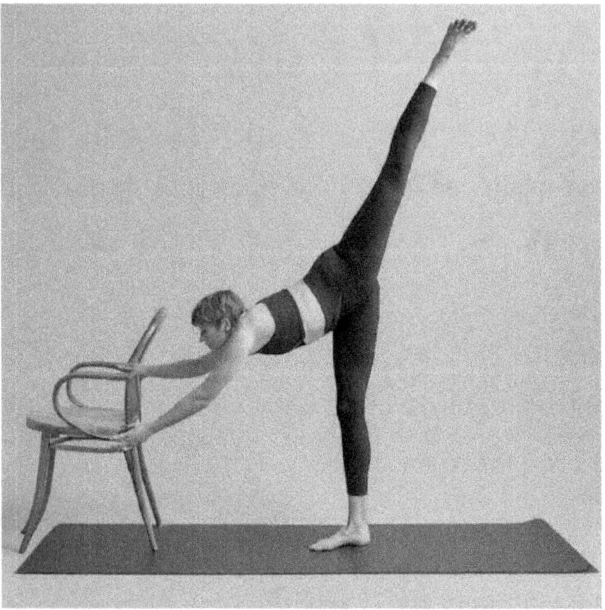

Benefits: Increases heart rate, strengthens quadriceps and core, activates pelvic floor indirectly.

Tips: Keep your back straight and core engaged throughout the movement. Don't lift your knees too high if you have knee issues.

Sets & Reps: 3 sets of 30-60 seconds each.

9. SEATED KNEE TO CHEST PULL:

Introduction: This gentle exercise stretches the lower back and hip flexors, indirectly improving pelvic floor flexibility.

Instructions:

-Sit upright in a chair with your back straight and feet flat on the floor.

-Hug one knee to your chest, engaging your core. Hold for 10-15 seconds, then slowly release.

-Repeat with the other leg.

-Continue for 5-10 repetitions per leg.

Illustration:

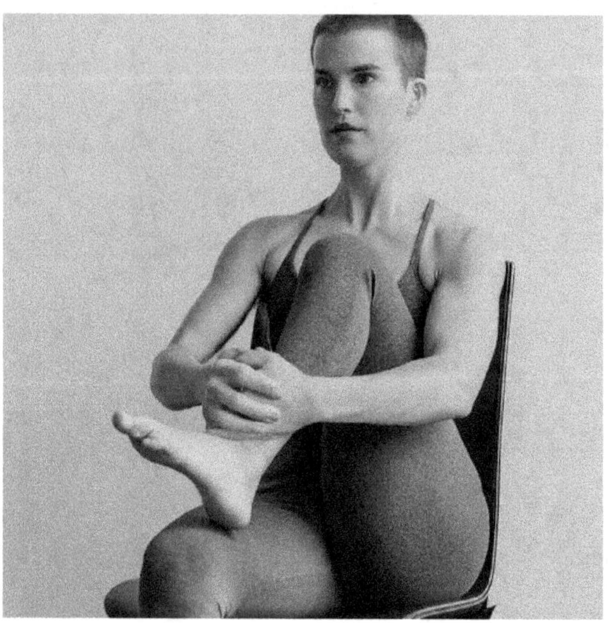

Benefits: Stretches lower back and hip flexors, improves flexibility, and helps relax muscles.

Tips: Breathe deeply throughout the stretch. Don't force anything that causes pain.

Sets & Reps: 3 sets of 5-10 repetitions per leg.

10. Modified Butterfly Stretch:

Introduction: This stretch opens the inner thighs and hips, promoting relaxation and indirectly impacting pelvic floor flexibility.

Instructions:

-Sit upright in a chair with your back straight and feet flat on the floor.

-Bring the soles of your feet together in front of you, letting your knees fall outwards as far as comfortable.

-Gently press your knees down with your hands, engaging your core and maintaining a straight back. Hold for 10-15 seconds, then release.

-Repeat 5-10 times.

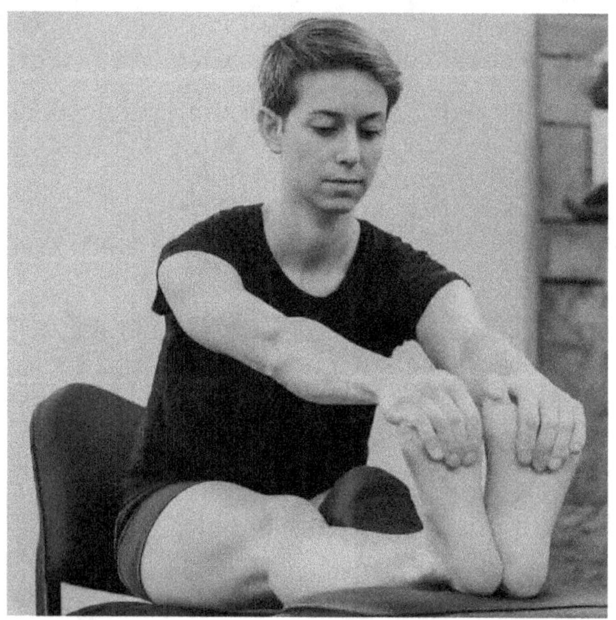

Benefits: Stretches inner thighs and hips, improves flexibility, and promotes relaxation.

Tips: Don't force the stretch beyond your comfort level. Listen to your body and stop if you feel any pain.

Sets & Reps: 3 sets of 5-10 repetitions.

CONCLUSION:

As you turn the final page, remember this book isn't the end of your pelvic floor journey, but rather the Launchpad. You've unlocked the potential of your chair, transforming it into a tool for strengthening, empowering, and reconnecting with your pelvic floor.

Think back to where you began. Perhaps there were anxieties about bladder control, pelvic pain, or simply a desire for improved core stability. You've learned that small, chair-assisted exercises can lead to big changes, proving that progress isn't just achievable, it's accessible.

This isn't a goodbye, but a "see you soon." Remember, these exercises are just the beginning. As you progress, explore variations, challenge yourself with new movements, and even incorporate other forms of exercise. Let your chair remain your companion, but remember, your body is capable of even more.

This journey isn't just about strengthening muscles; it's about empowering yourself. With each squeeze, lift, and breath, you cultivate confidence, awareness, and a deeper understanding of your body's incredible potential. Remember, a strong pelvic floor doesn't just improve physical well-being; it supports a vibrant, active life.

You're not alone on this path. Join the thriving community of individuals who understand the power of pelvic floor health. Share your successes, connect with others, and inspire them to embark on their own journeys. Let your progress be a testament to the effectiveness of these exercises and the power of community support.

As a professional dedicated to pelvic floor health, I'd be incredibly grateful if you could share your experience with a 5-star review. Your feedback helps me reach others seeking similar guidance and empowers them to take charge of their well-being.

So, dear reader, remember, your chair can be more than just a seat; it can be a gateway to a stronger, healthier, and more empowered you. Continue your journey, explore its possibilities, and share your passion with the world. May your pelvic floor health continue to flourish, one controlled movement at a time.